I0697459

EVERYTHING ABOUT DUKAN DIET

Complete Nutritional Cookbook, Foods, Meal Plan And Recipes To Unlock Your Weight Loss Journey For Lasting Results

DR. ALVIN BRANTLEY

© 2023 ALVIN BRANTLEY

All rights reserved. No part of this book may be reproduced, stored, or transmitted in any form or by any means, electronic, mechanical, photocopying, recording, scanning, or otherwise, without the prior written permission of the author.

Disclaimer

The information provided in this book is intended for general informational purposes only. It is not a substitute for professional medical advice, diagnosis, or treatment.

You should not use the information in this book for diagnosing or treating a health problem or disease by self decision. Always seek the advice of your physician or other qualified health provider with any questions you may have regarding a medical condition.

The author and publisher of this book make no representations or warranties with respect to the accuracy, applicability, fitness, or completeness of the contents of this book. The information contained in this book is based on the author's research and experience, and it is shared with the understanding that the author is not engaged in rendering medical, health, or any other kind of professional advice for you by this book.

The author does not endorse or promote any specific products, brands, or companies related to the contents provided in this book.

Any mention of products or services in this book is for informational purposes only and does not constitute an endorsement.

The author has not entered into any affiliate marketing agreements and has not signed any endorsement deals with individuals, organizations, or companies.

Readers are encouraged to consult with their healthcare providers before making any dietary or lifestyle chaSnges based on the information provided in this book. The author and publisher disclaim any liability for the decisions made by readers based on the information in this book.

Contents

Knowledge About The Dukan Diet

Dr. Pierre Dukan, a French nutritionist, created the well-known Dukan Diet, a weight-loss regimen that became well-known throughout the world for its unusual methodology and alleged efficacy. This diet prioritizes the consumption of lean protein and is designed around a set of principles and a phased strategy to help promote lasting weight loss.

CHAPTER ONE

The Dukan Diet's History

Early in the new millennium, Dr. Pierre Dukan developed the Dukan Diet, based on his encounters with patients looking for efficient and sustainable weight loss methods.

Following the release of Dr. Dukan's book "The Dukan Diet," which provided a detailed description of the regimen, the diet gained widespread recognition.

The strategy gained popularity because it was straightforward, placing an emphasis on whole meals rather than calculating calories.

Fundamentals And Philosophies

The idea behind the Dukan Diet is to include meals that are high in protein and low in carbohydrates in one's regular diet. Limiting carbs and fats while consuming lean protein sources including fish, fowl, and tofu is recommended by the diet. It also promotes the consumption of oat bran, an essential ingredient thought to facilitate digestion and enhance the overall effectiveness of the diet.

The Dukan Diet Has Four Phases

The Dukan Diet is divided into four main stages, each of which has a different function in the process of losing weight. The Attack Phase, Cruise Phase, Consolidation Phase, and Stabilization

Phase are these stages. Different foods and guidelines are introduced at each phase to help participants lose weight gradually and sustainably.

Phase of Attack

The Attack Phase, the initial stage, is distinguished by a focus on consuming just pure protein. Participants are encouraged to consume any amount of lean protein sources they choose during this phase. This phase, which usually lasts for a brief period, aims to induce ketosis, which will accelerate weight reduction.

Cruise Section

The Cruise Phase, which comes after the Attack Phase, keeps the focus on protein while introducing vegetables into the diet.

Days of pure protein and days of protein mixed with specific vegetables alternate during this period. The sequence of alternating steps continues until the targeted weight loss objectives are met.

Phase of Consolidation

The transition to a more varied and balanced diet occurs during the Consolidation Phase.

It emphasizes protein consumption while progressively introducing other dietary groups including fruits, dairy, and entire grains.

This stage assists the body in adjusting to a more sustainable eating routine and attempts to prevent sudden weight gain.

Phase of Stabilization

The goal of the last stage, stabilization, is to keep the weight loss that has been accomplished.

It is recommended that participants maintain a well-balanced diet and apply the knowledge gained from the earlier stages to their long-term way of living. Sustained success on the Dukan Diet depends on consistent commitment to its principles.

CHAPTER TWO

Crucial Advantages And Success Stories

Many people have stated that the Dukan Diet has been beneficial in helping them lose weight. It is thought that focusing on foods high in protein and using a systematic strategy will help manage weight in the short and long terms. Success stories about the diet frequently emphasize how well it works to lessen cravings, increase satiety, and create a positive relationship with food.

Individual outcomes may differ, so before making any big dietary adjustments, it's important to take into account any preexisting medical conditions and speak with a healthcare provider.

First Things First

Careful planning is necessary before starting the Dukan Diet to guarantee a smooth and fruitful trip toward your weight loss objectives. The first steps are learning the basics of the diet plan and implementing necessary lifestyle changes.

How To Be Ready For The Dukan Diet

It's important to evaluate your existing eating habits and level of mental preparedness for a major nutritional shift before beginning the Dukan Diet. Learning about the four unique phases of the diet—Attack, Cruise, Consolidation, and Stabilization—and designing a plan that fits your preferences and lifestyle are the first steps in preparing for the diet.

Food Purchasing

Careful grocery shopping is essential to following the Dukan Diet. Dietary success can be achieved by understanding what foods are permitted and organizing your meals accordingly. Because the diet focuses on lean protein, specific vegetables, and low fat, it's important to know what foods are permitted so you can shop wisely.

Kitchen Requirements

Having the right supplies and equipment in your kitchen is crucial to a successful Dukan Diet. Having the right kitchen basics improves your ability to follow the diet's requirements, from choosing the best cooking oils to purchasing a food scale for accurate portion control.

Having Reasonable Objectives

Setting realistic goals is an essential part of the Dukan Diet. Setting reasonable goals helps people maintain motivation during different diet periods. This entails being aware of the fundamentals of the diet and realizing how crucial it is to lose weight gradually and sustainably.

How To Determine True Weight

The idea of "True Weight," a tailored weight goal that takes into account variables like age, exercise level, and medical history, is one distinctive feature of the Dukan Diet. A healthier and more achievable weight loss journey is encouraged by calculating your True Weight, which gives you a realistic goal to strive towards.

Evaluating Your Preparedness

It's important to determine whether you're ready for the challenges and adjustments that come with the Dukan Diet before committing wholeheartedly. This entails assessing your way of life, your network of support, and your dedication to implementing the required changes.

To ensure long-term success with the Dukan Diet, assessing preparedness is an essential first step.

CHAPTER THREE

Assacred Stage

Dr. Pierre Dukan, a French nutritionist, created the well-known Dukan Diet, a weight-loss program that is divided into four phases, the first of which is called the Attack Phase.

This phase appeals to people who are ready to see results right away because it is marked by a rapid and large reduction in weight.

The Attack Phase: What Is It?

The Dukan Diet's Attack Phase is designed to help people lose weight quickly by following a high-protein, low-carbohydrate diet. The main goal of this phase, which usually lasts two to seven days, is to accelerate the metabolism and start burning fat. The Dukan Diet's Attack Phase is when adherents concentrate on eating foods high in lean protein and low in fat and carbohydrates.

Foods Permitted And Prohibited

A detailed list of permitted and prohibited foods defines the Attack Phase. Lean proteins are the main attraction; lean chicken, fish, eggs, and beef cuts are all recommended. These protein sources minimize the consumption of fats and carbohydrates while giving the body the fuel it needs. Conversely, during this phase, foods high in fat and carbohydrates are strictly prohibited. Later on in the diet, vegetables are progressively added back in, despite being restricted.

Meal Plans For Attack Phase Samples

During the Attack Phase, putting together a healthy and productive food plan is essential to success. A range of lean proteins, including grilled chicken, turkey, and fish, are frequently included in sample meal plans.

Non-starchy veggies are frequently included with these meals, which helps to supply important nutrients while limiting the amount of carbohydrates consumed. To make sure that adherents obtain enough nourishment without going over their daily protein allowance, portion control is stressed.

Success Advice

Although the Dukan Diet's Attack Phase can result in quick weight loss, success depends on following specific rules. It's critical to stay hydrated because a high-protein diet may cause more water loss.

The efficiency of the diet can be further increased by including physical activity, even in modest amounts. In addition, choosing lean, high-quality proteins and exercising portion control is crucial for establishing and sustaining success throughout the Attack Phase. By implementing these suggestions, you can facilitate a more seamless progression into the later stages of the Dukan Diet and create the conditions for long-term weight loss.

CHAPTER FOUR

Cruise Section

Dr. Pierre Dukan, a French dietitian, developed the well-known Dukan Diet, a four-phase weight-loss program. The diet's second phase, after the Attack Phase, is called the Cruise Phase. This phase emphasizes lean proteins while adding more meals to the diet to achieve sustainable and steady weight loss.

How To Handle The Cruise Phase

As was decided upon in the Attack Phase, people continue to eat an infinite amount of lean protein during the Cruise Phase. The main characteristic of this phase, though, is the switching between days when non-starchy veggies are reintroduced and days when just protein is consumed. This substitution is meant to provide the diet with some variety while still providing necessary vitamins and minerals.

Increasing Food Options

Increasing the variety of food options available beyond what was permitted during the Attack Phase is one of the main objectives of the Cruise Phase.

Apart from lean proteins like fish and poultry, people can also include a range of non-starchy veggies in their meals. This expansion helps create a more balanced and nutrient-dense eating plan in addition to making the diet more maintainable.

Making Well-Composed Meals

The focus during the Cruise Phase is on preparing meals that are balanced and include both non-starchy veggies and lean proteins. This method guarantees that people get more fiber, vitamins, and minerals, among other nutrients. Changing up the food options makes the diet more pleasant and easier to stick to for a longer amount of time, which helps people lose weight over the long run.

Progress Tracking And Modifications

Like any weight loss regimen, the key to success is keeping track of your progress. People are urged to measure themselves, keep track of their weight reduction, and evaluate how their clothes fit during the

Cruise Phase of the Dukan Diet. Adjustments can be made, including extending protein-only days or upping physical activity, if weight reduction stalls or plateaus. This adaptability enables a customized weight reduction strategy and aids in overcoming obstacles for each person.

The Dukan Diet's Cruise Phase represents a change toward a more diverse and long-term eating schedule.

People can lose weight steadily and consistently by emphasizing balanced meals and including non-starchy vegetables. Ensuring that the diet stays successful and customizable to meet personal needs and preferences requires regular progress monitoring and appropriate adjustments.

Slowly Introducing Novel Foods

Dieters can reintroduce some of the foods that were banned in the earlier phases during the consolidation phase.

This gradual introduction makes eating more varied and pleasurable while preventing weight gain that happens too quickly. Fruits, whole grains, and some dairy products bring diversity to the diet and increase its long-term sustainability.

Duration And Rules

The amount of weight lost during the early phases determines how long the consolidation phase lasts.

The general rule of thumb is to allow five days for each pound lost during the Cruise Phase. But to make sure the body adjusts to the adjustments and stabilizes the weight loss, Dr. Dukan advises waiting at least ten days. To get the most out of the Consolidation Phase, you must follow these instructions.

CHAPTER FIVE

Techniques For Sustaining Loss Of Weight

People are urged to use tactics that support maintaining the weight loss they had attained in the earlier phases during the consolidation phase.

An effective plan must include these essential components: eating a high-protein diet, exercising frequently, and drinking plenty of water. These habits help you live a healthier lifestyle and help your body maintain the weight loss you've achieved over time.

Finding A Happy-Go-Body Discipline

The Dukan Diet's emphasis on striking a balance between fun and discipline is one of its distinctive features. The Consolidation Phase permits greater flexibility in eating, in contrast to the prior phases that emphasize tight rules. Maintaining a healthy relationship with food, avoiding feelings of deprivation, and raising the chances of long-term success in weight management all depend on this balance.

A pivotal point in the weight-loss process is the Dukan Diet's Consolidation Phase. It makes it easier to gradually reintroduce a range of meals, making weight management more fun and sustainable.

Following the suggested principles and implementing useful tactics can help people move into a phase that strikes a balance between fun and discipline, which will ultimately help them maintain their weight over the long run.

Phase Of Stabilization

An essential part of the Dukan Diet, which is meant to support people in maintaining their weight loss over time, is the Stabilization Phase. The Stabilization Phase of the diet places more emphasis on creating lifelong behaviors to avoid gaining back weight than the earlier phases, which concentrate on quick weight loss.

Creating Long-Term Habits

Strict food restrictions are less important during the stabilization phase and more focus is placed on developing durable lifestyle modifications.

The idea is to incorporate healthier routines into day-to-day activities so that maintaining a healthy weight becomes second nature. During this stage, people are encouraged to eat in a reasonable, balanced manner while continuing to be conscious of the foods they choose.

Guidelines For The Phase Of Stabilization

A set of guidelines is introduced during the stabilization phase to help people keep up their weight loss. These guidelines include a weekly "pure protein" day, moderate physical activity, and a gradual return of previously banned foods. People can discover a sustainable and pleasurable eating pattern that helps them maintain their weight by progressively reintroducing a greater range of foods.

Honoring Your Achievement

It's important to pause and recognize weight loss accomplishments as people enter the Stabilization Phase. Rewarding oneself for the effort put in to achieve their ideal weight can inspire someone to stick with their healthy lifestyle. During this stage, people are encouraged to take stock of their journey, acknowledging the improvements they have made and how they have affected their general well-being.

Handling Obstacles

Recognizing that obstacles are an inevitable part of any long-term path, the Dukan Diet offers suggestions for overcoming difficulties during the Stabilization Phase.

Whether it's a brief increase in weight or a break from long-standing routines, this stage highlights the value of resilience and an optimistic outlook.

People who see failures as teaching opportunities are better able to overcome obstacles and keep moving forward in their quest for long-term weight maintenance.

the Dukan Diet's Stabilization Phase signifies the change from a rigorous weight-loss program to the development of long-lasting habits.

It offers a road plan for people to successfully navigate their post-diet lives, guaranteeing the long-term advantages attained during the earlier stages.

People can develop a balanced and healthy lifestyle that supports their weight management objectives by following the guidelines, celebrating their accomplishments, and remaining resilient in the face of adversity.

Menus For The Dukan Diet

A big part of the Dukan Diet is eating meals high in protein. Fish, poultry, and lean meats are frequently used in dishes. Inspiring recipes highlight protein in inventive ways that guarantee adherence to the diet's tenets while maintaining a tasty and fulfilling dinner.

Attack Phase Cookbooks

Meals during the Attack Phase mostly consist of sources of lean protein. Fish fillets, stir-fried lean beef, and grilled chicken breast are some foods that you might try during this time.

These dishes are meant to be varied yet still follow the limited food list for this first stage.

Cruise Phase Cookbooks

Recipes grow more varied as the diet advances to the Cruise Phase, including lean proteins and certain vegetables. Turkey lettuce wraps, fish with steamed veggies, and veggie and chicken skewers are a few examples of recipes for this phase.

These recipes demonstrate the range and adaptability that can be attained during the Cruise Phase.

Recipes For The Consolidation Phase

Reintroducing more food groups is permitted during the consolidation phase, and dishes make use of this increased diversity. Fruit salads, whole grain pasta with veggies, and cheese and legume meals are a few examples of recipes. The goal of these meals is to maintain weight while offering a range of nutrients.

Recipes For The Stabilization Phase

Recipes adopt a more flexible approach during the stabilization phase, using a variety of meals and placing an emphasis on portion management and a balanced diet.

Quinoa salads, well-balanced stir-fries, and dishes that combine a variety of lean proteins, veggies, and complete grains are a few examples of recipe ideas.

Sample Menus For Every Stage

For every stage of the Dukan Diet, for example, meal plans are supplied to help with actual implementation.

These programs provide direction on daily food consumption, assisting people in navigating dietary complexities and making wise decisions.

Every meal plan is designed to fit the unique needs and constraints of the associated phase, guaranteeing a methodical and efficient approach to weight loss and maintenance.

CHAPTER SIX

Advice And Detection

The Dukan Diet has its share of difficulties, just like every diet. It is critical to recognize potential hazards and have contingency plans to avoid them. Plateaus, dietary monotony, and social circumstances are common problems. Placing a brief return to the Attack Phase or modifying the protein-to-vegetable ratio can help overcome plateaus.

Keeping the diet interesting and fun requires experimenting with different protein and vegetable combinations to fight boredom.

To stay on course in social circumstances, preparation and communication may be necessary.

Remaining Inspired

Sustaining motivation is essential during the Dukan Diet process. Maintaining motivation can be facilitated by establishing reasonable objectives, monitoring advancement, and acknowledging successes of whatever size. Finding a network of friends, family, or online communities to lean on also offers accountability and motivation.

Rewarding achievement of milestones with something other than food helps to promote positive behavior.

Combining Exercise

Although the Dukan Diet mostly focuses on dietary adjustments, including exercise improves general health and helps with weight management.

Dr. Dukan advises introducing exercise gradually and adjusting for each person's degree of fitness.

Exercises that enhance the diet, such as walking, cycling, or strength training, encourage a holistic approach to wellness.

Sample Menus For Every Stage

Making healthy, filling meals is essential to following the Dukan Diet. Meal plan examples can serve as a source of ideas and direction.

Meals during the Attack Phase may consist of non-fat dairy, eggs, and lean meats.

Vegetables are added during the Cruise Phase, making a variety of salads and stir-fries possible.

While fruits, healthy grains, and celebratory meals are included in the Consolidation Phase, the Permanent Stabilization Phase places more emphasis on a varied and balanced diet to ensure long-term success.

the Dukan Diet emphasizes protein-rich foods and gradually reintroduces other food groups, providing a systematic and progressive approach to weight loss.

Even though many people find success with them, it's crucial to speak with a healthcare provider before beginning any diet.

Individuals can enhance their odds of long-term weight maintenance and traverse the Dukan Diet more easily by comprehending the phases, eliminating obstacles, and applying success strategies.

Discussing Common Mistakes:

The Dukan Diet has drawn criticism and misconceptions despite its widespread appeal. One such myth is that it ignores other vital nutrients in favor of relying only on meat consumption. As it happens, the diet encourages a variety of protein sources, such as dairy, plant-based proteins, and lean meats. It's not an all-meat diet; rather, protein is deliberately emphasized.

Myth: Inadequate Nutrient Balance: Detractors frequently claim that the Dukan Diet is inadequate in terms of nutrients and can result in dietary deficits. Later stages of the diet, however, include a wider range of foods, guaranteeing a more complete nutrient intake. Adding fruits, vegetables, and whole grains later on helps create a well-rounded nutritional profile.

misunderstanding: Unsustainability: The sustainability of the Dukan Diet is the subject of another misunderstanding. Critics contend that it is not long-term sustainable due to the early phases' restrictions. However, the goal of the Stabilization phase's emphasis on lifestyle modifications and the subsequent phases' progressive reintroduction of foods is to create enduring, healthful eating habits.

Myth: Rapid Weight Loss Solution: There is a misconception among certain people that the Dukan Diet is a rapid weight loss solution. The effectiveness of the diet depends on sustained dedication, even though the early stages may result in quick weight loss. The later stages focus on eating a balanced, diverse diet and engaging in regular physical activity to maintain a healthy weight.

Myth: Risk of Kidney Damage: There have been questions about how a diet heavy in protein may affect the health of the kidneys. There is, however, little evidence linking high-protein diets, such as Dukan, to kidney injury. Before starting such diets, people with pre-existing kidney issues should speak with a healthcare provider.

Myth: One-Size-Fits-All strategy: According to critics, the Dukan Diet ignores individual variances in favor of a one-size-fits-all strategy. The diet is flexible, allowing people to modify it to fit their nutritional needs and preferences while still adhering to the recommended standards, even though the fundamental concepts stay the same.

Conclusion

with its four-phase strategy, the Dukan Diet provides an organized method for losing weight. Although it has drawn criticism as well as praise, clearing out common misconceptions is essential for a comprehensive understanding.

The Dukan Diet seeks to offer a long-term, sustainable route to weight control by stressing long-term lifestyle modifications, progressively reintroducing foods, and concentrating on a range of protein sources. Those who are thinking about adopting this diet should speak with medical experts to be sure it fits their unique needs.

BEYOND THE DIET: Although the Dukan Diet offers a methodical way to lose weight, its effects extend beyond the scale. The diet places a strong emphasis on developing a positive relationship with food, encouraging mindful eating practices, and advancing long-term well-being.

Post-Diet Maintenance: For many people, maintaining their weight loss is a major challenge. The Dukan Diet's post-diet maintenance phase acknowledges this and provides advice on maintaining the gains made. Maintaining a healthy weight can be facilitated by including regular exercise, controlling portion sizes, and continuing to emphasize meals high in protein.

Creating a Healthier Lifestyle:

People can create a healthier lifestyle with the help of the Dukan Diet. After the suggested phases are over, followers are urged to develop routines like consistent exercise, drinking enough water, and getting enough sleep. These lifestyle changes improve people's general well-being and assist them in adopting a sustainable and balanced approach to health.

Additional Health Benefits: The Dukan Diet is linked to several health advantages despite being primarily intended for weight loss. Prioritizing lean proteins can help maintain muscle mass, and cutting less on processed carbs may have a beneficial effect on blood sugar levels. Furthermore, the diet's emphasis on whole, nutrient-dense foods enhances dietary intake and general wellness.

the Dukan Diet offers a thorough approach to health and wellness, going beyond a short-term weight loss solution. The stages that are designed offer a way to lose weight, but the diet's core ideas—like emphasizing protein and practicing mindful eating—can be incorporated into a long-term, sustainable way of life. As with any diet, it's best to speak with medical professionals to ensure safe, customized weight management.

www.ingramcontent.com/pod-product-compliance
Lightning Source LLC
Chambersburg PA
CBHW060811260726
48660CB00002B/888